BLOOD '

A+ DIET BOOK

"100+ Delicious and Nutritious Recipes to Aid Optimal Wellness and Achieve Optimal Health for Your Blood Type"

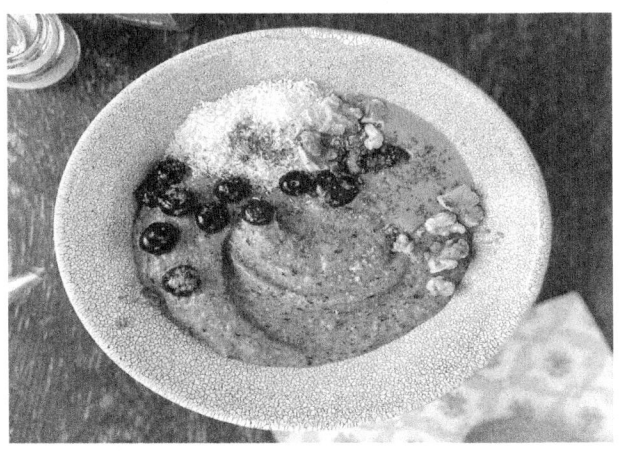

Dayna G. Murphy

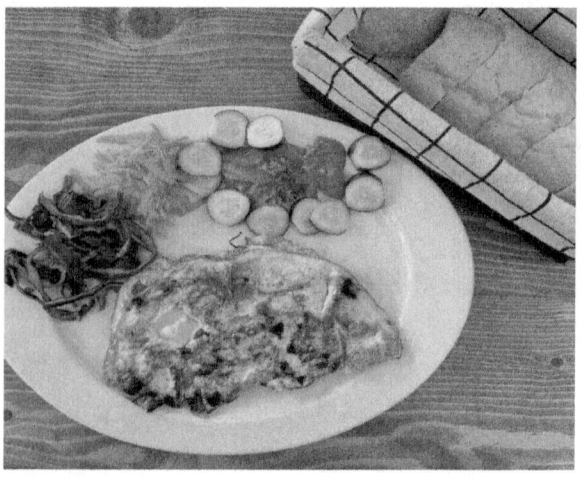

Table of Contents

INTRODUCTION

My friend Michael has an A+ blood type, and he struggled with finding the right foods to keep him healthy. When he started following the recipes in my A+ diet book, something amazing happened. He began to feel better, with more energy and fewer health problems. This inspired me to write and share the correct diet with others.

Seeing the positive changes in Michael's life made me realize the power of eating right for your blood type. The book not only helped him but also gave me the motivation to help more people like him. It's incredible how the right foods can make such a big difference. Now, I'm on a mission to share this knowledge with as many people as possible, so they can experience the same positive changes in their lives. Michael's story is a testament to the impact of the A+ diet on our health and well-being.

Welcome to the full A+ Blood Type Diet guide. This book will help you grasp the significant relationship between your blood type and the foods you eat, allowing you to live a happier, more vibrant life. Whether you're new to the notion or want to brush up on your knowledge, this book will provide you with insights, techniques, and scrumptious recipes that correspond to the dietary preferences of people with blood type A+.

The A+ Blood Type Diet is more than simply a diet; it's a way of life suited to your specific physiological needs. Throughout this book, you will learn about the basics of blood type determination, the effects of ABO and Rh factors, and how your specific blood type might affect your health and well-being.

Learn how to use food as medicine, with a focus on advantageous food groups, suggested fruits and vegetables, and high-quality protein sources. Discover which foods to limit or remove, as well the significance of lectins in your diet.

This book provides practical suggestions and sample meal plans on anything from creating balanced meals to dining out smartly. Dive into delectable A+ diet recipes that not only suit your blood type but also your taste buds. This book is your key to becoming a healthier, more vibrant version of yourself. It's time to embark on a path to wellness, armed with the A+ Blood Type Diet knowledge.

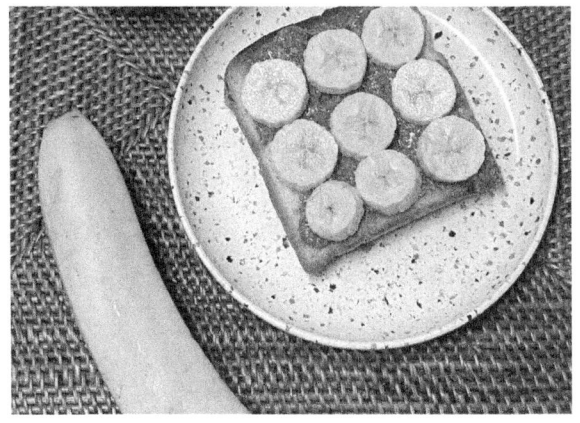

CHAPTER 1

Understanding the A+ Blood Type

The Fundamentals of Blood Types

The presence or absence of particular antigens on the surface of red blood cells determines blood type, which is a key feature of human biology. The ABO system is the most well-known blood type classification system, and it divides people into four blood types: A, B, AB, and O. The ABO system is based on whether or not two antigens, A and B, are present.

- **Blood Type A:** Individuals with blood type A carry the A antigen on their red blood cells.
- **Blood Type B:** People with blood type B have the B antigen.
- **Blood Type AB:** Individuals with blood type AB have A and B antigens.
- **Blood Type O:** Individuals with blood type O lack both the A and B antigens.

Aside from the ABO system, another key blood type characteristic is the Rh factor (Rhesus factor). It may be Rh-positive (+) or Rh-negative (-).

Blood types influence medical practices such as blood transfusions and organ transplantation. A person with blood type A, for example, can usually get blood from type A or type O donors but not from type B or type AB donors. The presence or absence of particular antibodies in the recipient's plasma causes this compatibility.

The Health Consequences of Blood Type A+

Blood type A+ is distinguished by the presence of A antigens on the surface of red blood cells as well as the presence of the Rh factor (Rh-positive). Although blood type does not affect general health, it has been suggested that it may influence some health variables and predispositions.

Some of the potential health consequences of blood type A+ include:

- **Cardiovascular Health:** According to some research, people with blood type A may be at a slightly increased risk of cardiovascular disorders such as heart disease and stroke. A heart-healthy diet and lifestyle are critical for mitigating this risk.

- **Digestive Health:** People with blood type A may be more prone to digestive disorders. As a result, the Blood Type Diet was created, which advises particular dietary restrictions customized to each blood type.

- **Immunity:** Immune function and susceptibility to some infections may be affected by blood type A+. More research, however, is required to completely comprehend these linkages.

While these correlations exist, individual health is determined by a complex combination of genetic, behavioral, and environmental variables. Blood type should not be used as the sole determinant of health decisions, and interaction with healthcare specialists is required for customized health management.

The Relationship Between Blood Type and Diet

The blood type diet concept claims that an individual's nutritional choices should be determined by their blood type. Specific blood types emerged at different points in human history and are better suited to distinct diets, according to the theory.

The recommended diet for people with blood type A+ often includes:

- **Plant-Based Diets**: A diet high in fruits, vegetables, and whole grains is frequently recommended. These meals are thought to be better tolerated and offer vital nutrients for people with blood type A+.

- **Lean Protein:** Consumption of animal protein is limited, with an emphasis on lean sources such as poultry and fish. It is frequently recommended that red meat be consumed in moderation.

- **Avoidance of some Foods**: The diet advises against or limits the consumption of dairy products and some high-fat meats. Furthermore, people with blood type A+ are often recommended to reduce their intake of lectin-containing foods because they are thought to be less well-tolerated.

CHAPTER 2: THE SCIENCE BEHIND THE A+ DIET

Genetics and Blood Type

How Is My Blood Type Determined?

The presence or absence of certain antigens on the surface of red blood cells determines blood type. These antigens are passed down via families, and their combination determines an individual's blood type. The ABO system and the Rh factor are the two basic blood group systems used to determine blood type.

1. ABO Blood Group System: The ABO Blood Group System divides blood types into four major groups: A, B, AB, and O. The presence or absence of two antigens on the surface of red blood cells - antigen A and antigen B - determines this categorization. These antigen-producing genes are inherited from one's parents.

- Individuals with blood type AB inherit an A antigen from one parent and a B antigen from the other.
- If a person inherits two A antigens, they will be of blood type A.
- They will have blood type B if they inherit two B antigens.
- Individuals with blood type O will inherit two O (no antigen) genes.

2. Rh Factor (also known as Rhesus Factor): The Rh factor, in addition to the ABO blood group system, is an important component in blood typing. The Rh factor is a protein that can be Rh-positive (+) or Rh-negative (-) on the surface of red blood cells. The presence or absence of this protein determines an individual's Rh status.

- Individuals that have the Rh factor on their red blood cells are Rh-positive (e.g., A+ or B+).
- They are Rh-negative (e.g., A- or B-) if they lack the Rh factor.

The ABO blood group and the Rh factor are commonly used to express blood type. Someone with A antigens and the Rh factor, for example, has blood type A+, whereas someone with B antigens but no Rh factor has blood type B-.

The Function of ABO and Rh Factors

The ABO blood type system and the Rh factor are important in many areas of medicine, including transfusion medicine and organ transplantation:

1. Blood Transfusions: It is critical to match the donor's blood type to the recipient's blood type in order to avoid serious responses when receiving a blood transfusion. Incompatible blood types can cause hemolysis, a potentially fatal disorder in which the recipient's immune system assaults and kills the transfused red blood cells. As a result, a person with blood type A can safely receive blood from donors with blood types A or O, but not from donors with blood types B or AB, and the Rh factor must also be compatible.

2. **Organ Transplantation:** Blood type compatibility is an important consideration in organ transplantation. To reduce the chance of organ rejection, organs like as the heart, kidney, and liver must be matched as closely as possible to the recipient's blood type.

3. **Pregnancy and Rh Incompatibility:** Rh incompatibility between the mother and the baby during pregnancy can result in hemolytic illness in the infant. When a Rh-negative woman carries a Rh-positive fetus, the mother's immune system responds by producing antibodies against the Rh factor. This disorder can be avoided by administering Rh immunoglobulin (RhIg) during pregnancy.

CHAPTER 2: EATING RIGHT FOR BLOOD TYPE A+

Food as Medicine

The Food as Medicine Hypothesis

The concept of *"food as medicine"* is a key tenet in nutrition and healthcare that emphasizes the importance of dietary choices in an individual's general health and well-being. This concept emphasizes the fact that the foods we eat can have an impact on our physical health, mental well-being, and susceptibility to various health disorders. It emphasizes the idea that a well-balanced and nutrient-dense diet can play an important role in sickness prevention and management. Here are some essential components of the food as medicine concept:

1. Nutrition and Healing: The foods we consume contain critical elements such as vitamins, minerals, antioxidants, and macronutrients such as carbs, proteins, and fats. These nutrients serve as the foundation of our bodies, aiding in cellular function, energy production, and immunological response.

2. Disease Prevention: A diet high in fruits, vegetables, whole grains, and lean proteins has been linked to a lower risk of chronic diseases such as heart disease, diabetes, and some malignancies. This emphasizes the preventive power of food decisions.

3. Managing Chronic disorders: Dietary changes can be an important aspect of treatment for those who have chronic health disorders like diabetes or hypertension. Proper nutrition can aid in the control of blood sugar levels, the reduction of blood pressure, and the prevention of problems.

4. Immunity and Inflammation: Certain foods have anti-inflammatory qualities and can help the immune system. A diet strong in processed and inflammatory foods, on the other hand, can contribute to chronic inflammation and impair the body's defenses.

5. Gut Health: The gastrointestinal system's health, especially the microbiome, is intimately related to general health. Diet alters gut bacteria composition, which affects digestion, metabolism, and the immune system.

6. Mental Health: New research suggests a link between food and mental health. Diets high in processed foods may raise the incidence of mood disorders, whereas nutrient-rich diets are related with reduced rates of sadness and anxiety.

Philosophy of the A+ Blood Type Diet

The A+ Blood Type Diet, is a nutritional philosophy that suggests an individual's blood type should dictate their food choices. For people with blood type A+, the diet philosophy stresses the following principles:

1. Plant-Based Priority: The A+ Blood Type Diet promotes the eating of a wide range of fruits and vegetables. It supports plant-based nutrition sources, highlighting that these foods are better suited to those with blood type A+.

2. Lean Protein: While it prefers plant-based proteins, it nevertheless allows for the addition of lean animal proteins like poultry and fish. Red meat should be ingested in moderation by persons with blood type A+.

3. Dairy and Grains: The diet recommends minimizing dairy products, especially for people who are lactose intolerant. It also recommends eating whole grains rather than processed grains.

4. Considerations for Lectins: One of the Blood Type Diet's unique aspects is its emphasis on lectins, which are proteins found in many foods. It argues that certain lectins may be intolerable to people with certain blood types and recommends avoiding these foods.

Foods to Embrace

Food Groups That Are Good For You

The A+ Blood Type Diet highlights numerous healthy food groups that are thought to be ideal for people with blood type A+. While it's important to approach this dietary philosophy with caution because the scientific data is weak, here are some food groups that are frequently advised as beneficial:

1. Fruits and Vegetables: Fruits and vegetables are high in important vitamins and minerals, as well as antioxidants and fiber. The diet promotes a wide variety of bright, fresh produce to offer essential nutrients while lowering the risk of chronic diseases.

2. Whole Grains: Whole grains like brown rice, quinoa, and oats include complex carbs that provide sustained energy as well as fiber for digestive health. Because of their nutritional value, these grains are frequently included in the A+ Blood Type Diet.

3. **Lean Proteins:** High-quality protein sources, both plant-based and animal-based, are encouraged. These proteins provide vital amino acids required for a variety of biological processes.

4. **Legumes:** Legumes, such as lentils, chickpeas, and black beans, are recommended for their high protein and fiber content. They are regarded as a good source of plant-based protein in the diet.

5. **Nuts and Seeds:** Nuts and seeds provide healthful fats, protein, and a variety of minerals. Because of their nutritious content, they can be consumed in moderation.

6. **Healthy Fats:** According to the diet, people with blood type A+ may benefit from healthy fats like avocados, olive oil, and fatty fish like salmon. These fats supply vital fatty acids and aid in general wellness.

Fruits and Vegetables to Eat

The A+ Blood Type Diet frequently advises certain fruits and vegetables for those with blood type A+. These options are thought to be more tolerable and to supply critical nutrients. Fruits and vegetables that are frequently suggested include:

- **Fruits:** Apples, berries (especially blueberries and cranberries), cherries, figs, and plums are examples of fruits. These fruits are regarded to be advantageous to those with blood type A+.
- **Vegetables:** Green, green vegetables such as kale and spinach are frequently recommended. Broccoli, carrots, and garlic are also regarded suitable options.

Sources of High-Quality Protein

Protein is a necessary macronutrient for the body, and the A+ Blood Type Diet recommends consuming high-quality protein sources. Protein sources for persons with blood type A+ are frequently recommended:

1. Poultry: Lean poultry, such as chicken and turkey, is a good source of protein for those with blood type A+.

2. Fish: For its high-quality protein and omega-3 fatty acids, certain forms of fish, such as salmon and trout, are recommended. These can be beneficial to both heart and brain health.

3. Plant-Based Proteins: Lentils and soy products such as tofu are marketed as plant-based protein sources. Protein can also be obtained from nuts and seeds such as almonds and flaxseeds.

4. Diary Alternatives: Dairy substitutes, such as soy milk and almond milk, may be preferred over regular dairy products, especially if lactose sensitivity is a concern.

Foods to Avoid

Items to Limit or Eliminate

The A+ Blood Type Diet philosophy suggests that individuals with blood type A+ may benefit from limiting or eliminating certain foods and food groups believed to be less compatible with their blood type. However, it's crucial to note that these recommendations are controversial, and the scientific evidence supporting these restrictions is limited. Here are some items often recommended to be limited or eliminated in the A+ Blood Type Diet:

1. Red Meat: The diet advises reducing the consumption of red meat, such as beef and lamb. This is based on the belief that red meat may not be well-tolerated by individuals with blood type A+ and could lead to various health issues.

2. Dairy Products: Dairy items, especially cow's milk, are often recommended to be limited or replaced with dairy alternatives due to the suggestion that lactose intolerance may be more common in individuals with blood type A+.

3. Processed and High-Fat Meats: Processed meats like bacon and sausages are often discouraged. High-fat meats, which are believed to be less compatible with blood type A+, are also advised to be consumed in moderation.

4. Certain Grains: The diet recommends avoiding or limiting wheat products, as they contain gluten. It suggests that gluten may be less well-tolerated by individuals with blood type A+. Rye and barley may also be restricted for the same reason.

5. Legumes: While some legumes are encouraged for their protein and fiber content, others, like lentils, are advised to be limited due to their lectin content (more on lectins below).

6. Processed and High-Sugar Foods: Processed and sugary foods are typically discouraged in most dietary philosophies. Reducing added sugars and processed foods is a general principle for overall health.

Foods That May Interfere with Your Health

The A+ Blood Type Diet suggests that some foods may interfere with the health of individuals with blood type A+. While these claims are not widely accepted within the medical community, the diet theory posits that certain foods may lead to digestive problems, inflammation, or other health issues in those with blood type A+. Foods that may be considered potential culprits include:

1. Lectin-Rich Foods: Lectins are proteins found in various foods, including grains, legumes, and some vegetables. The diet suggests that some lectins may be incompatible with blood type A+ and may lead to digestive discomfort and other health issues.

2. Dairy Products: Cow's milk and dairy products may be associated with digestive problems and discomfort in individuals with blood type A+ who are believed to have a higher likelihood of lactose intolerance.

3. Certain Grains: Grains that contain gluten, such as wheat, rye, and barley, are thought to be less well-tolerated by those with blood type A+. These grains may lead to digestive distress or inflammation.

4. High-Fat Meats: High-fat meats, especially red meat, are suggested to be less compatible with blood type A+ and may contribute to cardiovascular issues and other health problems.

The Impact of Lectins

Lectins are proteins found in various foods, including legumes, grains, and certain vegetables. The A+ Blood Type Diet theory suggests that lectins may have a negative impact on the health of individuals with blood type A+ by interfering with digestion and potentially contributing to inflammation and other health issues.

Lectins can bind to the lining of the gut and may interfere with the absorption of nutrients. However, it's essential to emphasize that the impact of lectins on health is a topic of ongoing research and debate in the scientific community. Most people can tolerate lectins without issues, and many lectin-containing foods are also highly nutritious.

CHAPTER 3: BLOOD TYPE A+ RECOMMENDED FOODS

1. MEAT AND POULTRY

Meat and Poultry	Suitable Choices	Portion Size	frequency per week
Chicken	Skinless chicken breast or thigh	4-6 oz (cooked)	2-3 times
Turkey	Lean turkey, especially breast meat	4-6 oz (cooked)	2-3 times
Lamb	Lean lamb cuts	4-6 oz (cooked)	2-3 times
Wild Game	Venison, rabbit, etc	4-6 oz (cooked)	2-3 times

Lean veal cuts	4-6 oz (cooked)	2-3 times

2. DIARY AND EGGS

Dairy and Eggs	Suitable Choices	Suggested Portion Size	frequency Per week
Yogurt	Plain, unsweetened yogurt	1 cup	2-4 times per week
Cheese	Feta, mozzarella, farmer cheese	1-2 ounces	2-4 times per week
Milk (if tolerated)	Soy or almond milk may be preferred	1 cup	2-4 times per week
Eggs	Eggs from cage-free or	2-3 eggs	2-4 times per week

	pastured hens		

3. SEAFOODS

Seafood	Suitable Choices	Portion Size	frequency Per week
Salmon	Salmon	4-6 oz (cooked)	2-3 times
Trout	Trout	4-6 oz (cooked)	2-3 times
Mackerel	Mackerel	4-6 oz (cooked)	2-3 times
Sardines	Sardines	4-6 oz (cooked)	2-3 times
Halibut	Halibut	4-6 oz (cooked)	2-3 times
Cod	Cod	4-6 oz (cooked)	2-3 times

,UTS AND SEEDS

Nuts and Seeds	Suitable Choices	Portion Size	frequency Per week
Almonds	Almonds	10-15 almonds	2-3 times
Walnuts	Walnuts	5-7 walnuts	2-3 times
Flaxseeds	Flaxseeds	About 1-2 tablespoons	2-3 times
Chia Seeds	Chia seeds	About 1-2 tablespoons	2-3 times
Pumpkin Seeds (Pepitas)	Pumpkin seeds (pepitas)	About 1-2 tablespoons	2-3 times
Sunflower Seeds	Sunflower seeds	About 1-2 tablespoons	2-3 times

5. GRAINS AND CEREALS

Grains and Cereals	Suitable Choices	Portion Size	frequency Per week
Oats	Rolled oats, steel-cut oats	About 1/2 to 1 cup (cooked)	2-3 times
Rice (Brown or Wild)	Brown rice, wild rice	About 1/2 to 1 cup (cooked)	2-3 times
Quinoa	Quinoa	About 1/2 to 1 cup (cooked)	2-3 times
Amaranth	Amaranth	About 1/2 to 1 cup (cooked)	2-3 times
Millet	Millet	About 1/2 to 1 cup (cooked)	2-3 times
Buckwheat	Buckwheat	About 1/2 to 1 cup (cooked)	2-3 times

J. BEVERAGES, TEAS AND COFFEE

Beverages, Teas, and Coffee	Suitable Choices	Portion Size	frequency Per week
Water	Water	8-10 glasses (8 oz)	Daily
Herbal Teas (e.g., chamomile, peppermint, ginger)	Herbal teas	As needed	3-4 times
Green Tea	Green tea	1-2 cups per day	3-4 times
Red Wine (if consumed)	Red Wine	Up to 5 oz (occasional)	Occasional

Coffee (if tolerated)	Black coffee (limit additives)	In moderation (1-2 cups per day)	Occasional

7. FRUITS

Fruits	Suitable Choices	Portion Size	frequency Per week
Apples	Apples	1 medium apple	3-4 times
Cherries	Cherries	1 cup	3-4 times
Plums	Plums	1 medium plum	3-4 times
Blueberries	Blueberries	1 cup	3-4 times
Papayas	Papayas	1/2 papaya	3-4 times
Pineapples	Pineapples	1 cup (cubed)	3-4 times

Plums (Red)	Red plums	1 medium red plum	3-4 times
Peaches	Peaches	1 medium peach	3-4 times
Elderberries	Elderberries	1 cup	3-4 times
Kiwi	Kiwi	1 medium kiwi	3-4 times
Pineapple Juice	Fresh pineapple juice	1 cup	3-4 times

8. HERBS AND SPICES

Herbs and Spices	Suitable Choices	Portion Size	frequency Per week
Basil	Basil	As needed for flavor	Regularly
Thyme	Thyme	As needed for flavor	Regularly

Rosemary	Rosemary	As needed for flavor	Regularly
Turmeric	Turmeric	As needed for flavor	Regularly
Parsley	Parsley	As needed for flavor	Regularly
Ginger	Ginger	As needed for flavor	Regularly

9. VEGETABLES

Vegetables	Suitable Choices	Portion Size	frequency Per week
Broccoli	Broccoli	1 cup (cooked)	3-4 times
Spinach	Spinach	1-2 cup (cooked)	3-4 times
Kale	Kale	1-2 cups (cooked)	3-4 times

Swiss Chard	Swiss chard	1-2 cups (cooked)	2-3 times
Collard Greens	Collard greens	1-2 cups (cooked)	2-3 times
Brussels Sprouts	Brussels sprouts	1 cup (cooked)	2-3 times
Carrots	Carrots	About 1 cup (cooked or raw)	2-3 times
Cabbage	Cabbage	1 cup (cooked)	2-3 times

10. BEANS AND LEGUMES

Beans and Legumes	Suitable Choices	Portion Size	frequency Per week
Black Eyed Peas	Black-eyed peas	½ to 1 cup (cooked)	2-3 times
Lentils	Lentils	½ to 1 cup (cooked)	3-4 times

Navy Beans	Navy beans	½ to 1 cup (cooked)	2-3 times
Adzuki Beans	Adzuki beans	½ to 1 cup (cooked)	2-3 times
Garbanzo Beans (Chickpeas)	Garbanzo beans (chickpeas)	½ to 1 cup (cooked)	2-3 times

11. OILS AND FATS

Oils and Fats	Suitable Choices	Portion Size	frequency Per week
Olive Oil	Extra virgin olive oil	As needed for cooking	Regularly
Flaxseed Oil	Cold-pressed flaxseed oil	As needed for dressing	Regularly

Walnut Oil	Walnut oil	As needed for dressing	Regularly
Canola Oil	Canola oil	As needed for cooking	Regularly
Avocado Oil	Avocado oil	As needed for cooking	Regularly

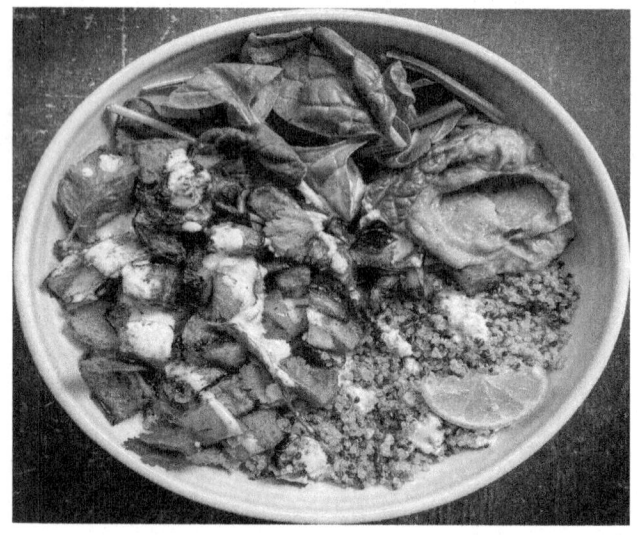

CHAPTER 4: RECIPES AND INGREDIENTS

Ten Breakfast Suggestions and How to Prepare them

1. Omelette with Vegetables

Ingredients:

- two huge eggs
- 1/4 cup bell peppers, chopped
- a quarter cup chopped tomatoes
- 1/4 cup chopped onions
- Season with salt and pepper to taste.
- Cooking with olive oil

Instructions: In a mixing dish, whisk together the eggs and season with salt and pepper. Melt a little olive oil in a nonstick skillet over medium heat. Sauté the diced vegetables for a few minutes, or until softened. Cook the omelette in half after pouring the whipped eggs over the vegetables. Cook for 1 minute more, or until the center is completely done. Serve immediately.

(Preparation time: 10 minutes)

2. Berry Smoothie Bowl

Ingredients:

- 1 cup mixed berries (blueberries, strawberries, etc.)
- a half banana
- 1 cup plain Greek yogurt (or dairy-free substitute)
- 2 tbsp of chia seeds
- **Optional:** 1 tablespoon honey or maple syrup
- **Toppings:** sliced almonds or shredded coconut

Instructions: In a blender, combine the berries, banana, Greek yogurt, and chia seeds until smooth. Fill a bowl halfway with the smoothie. If desired, drizzle with honey or maple syrup. Serve with sliced almonds or shredded coconut on top. Serve with a spoon.

(Preparation time: 5 minutes)

3. Banana Toast with Almond Butter

Ingredients:

- 2 slices whole-grain bread (A+ recommendation)
- two tbsp almond butter
- 1 sliced banana

- Optional cinnamon sprinkling

Instructions: Toast the whole-grain bread to your favorite crispness degree. Spread almond butter on each slice evenly. On top, arrange banana slices. If preferred, top with a pinch of cinnamon. Serve right away.

(Preparation time: 5 minutes)

4. Greek Yogurt Pudding

Ingredients:

- 1 cup plain Greek yogurt (or a dairy-free substitute)
- 1/2 cup berries, mixed
- 2 granola tablespoons
- **Optional:** 1 tablespoon honey or maple syrup

Instructions: Layer Greek yogurt, mixed berries, and granola in a glass or bowl. If desired, drizzle with honey or maple syrup.
Repeat for a second layer. With a spoon, serve.

(Preparation time: 5 minutes)

5. Poached Egg on Avocado Toast

Ingredients:

- 1 whole-grain bread slice

- mashed 1/2 ripe avocado
- 1 boiled egg
- Season with salt and pepper to taste.
- Optional red pepper flakes

Instructions: Toast the whole-grain bread to taste. On the toast, spread the mashed avocado. Serve with a poached egg on top. If desired, season with salt, pepper, and red pepper flakes. Serve right away.

(Preparation time: 15 minutes, including poaching the eggs)

6. Scrambled Spinach with Mushrooms

Ingredients:

- two huge eggs
- 1/2 cup spinach, chopped
- 1/4 cup mushrooms, sliced
- 1/4 cup chopped onions
- Cooking with olive oil
- Season with salt and pepper to taste.

Instructions: In a skillet over medium heat, heat the olive oil. Cook the onions and mushrooms until they soften. Cook until the spinach is wilted, about 5 minutes. Whisk the eggs with salt and pepper in a separate bowl. Pour the eggs and vegetables into the pan.

Cook, stirring gently, until the eggs are done to your liking. Serve immediately.
(Preparation time: 10 minutes)

7. Chia Seed Pudding

Ingredients:
- 2 tbsp of chia seeds
- 1 cup almond milk (or a dairy-free substitute)
- a half teaspoon of vanilla extract
- **Optional**: 1 tablespoon honey or maple syrup
- **Toppings**: sliced strawberries or other A+-friendly fruits

Instructions: Combine the chia seeds, almond milk, and vanilla essence in a mixing dish. If desired, sweeten with honey or maple syrup. Refrigerate overnight or for at least a few hours, stirring occasionally, until the mixture thickens. Serve with sliced strawberries or other fruit of your choice. Serve chilled.
(Preparation time: 5 minutes plus rest time)

8. Breakfast Bowl with Quinoa

Ingredients:

- 1 cooked cup quinoa
- 1 cup plain Greek yogurt (or dairy-free substitute)
- Peaches or other A+ fruits, sliced
- A smear of honey or maple syrup
- Almonds, chopped for crunch

Instructions: Layer cooked quinoa, Greek yogurt, and sliced peaches in a bowl.Drizzle with honey or maple syrup. Top with chopped almonds. Serve warm or cold for breakfast.

(Preparation time: 10 minutes if quinoa is already cooked)

9. Pancakes with an A+ rating

Ingredients:
- 1/2 cup spelt flour (A+ approved)
- a half teaspoon baking powder
- a quarter teaspoon of salt
- 1 cup almond milk (or dairy-free substitute)
- 1 tbsp honey (or maple syrup)
- 1 egg
- a smidgeon of vanilla extract
- Topping: fresh berries

Instructions: In a mixing basin, combine the spelt flour, baking powder, and salt. Mix almond milk, honey or maple syrup, egg, and vanilla essence in a separate basin. Stir together the wet and dry ingredients until smooth. Lightly oil a nonstick skillet over medium heat. To prepare pancakes, spoon little amounts of batter onto the pan. Cook until surface bubbles appear, then flip and cook until golden brown. Garnish with fresh berries.

(Preparation time: 15 minutes)

10. Wrap with sliced apple and nut butter
Ingredients:
- 1 whole-grain tortilla (A+ recommendation)
- 2 tbsp cashew or almond butter
- 1 finely sliced apple
- a dash of cinnamon

Instructions: In a dry skillet, warm the whole-grain tortilla gently. Cover the tortilla with the almond or cashew butter. Arrange the apple slices on top. For added flavor, sprinkle with cinnamon. Roll it up and eat it.

(Preparation time: 5 minutes)

Ten Lunch Suggestions and How to Prepare Them

1. Salad with Spinach and Chickpeas
Ingredients:
- 2 cups spinach leaves, fresh
- 1/2 cup chickpeas, cooked
- 1/4 cup cucumber, diced
- 1/4 cup red bell pepper, chopped
- 1/4 cup cherry tomatoes, sliced
- Dressing with olive oil and lemon juice
- Season with salt and pepper to taste.

Instructions: In a salad bowl, combine spinach, chickpeas, cucumber, red bell pepper, and cherry tomatoes. Season with salt and pepper and drizzle with olive oil and lemon juice. Serve chilled.
(Preparation time: 10 minutes)

2. Bowl of Quinoa with Roasted Vegetables
Ingredients:
- 1 cup quinoa, cooked
- roasted veggies (such as zucchini, bell peppers, and sweet potatoes)

- **Dressing:** olive oil and balsamic vinegar
- **Optional:** chopped fresh basil and crumbled feta cheese

Instructions: In a bowl, combine the cooked quinoa and roasted vegetables. Drizzle with balsamic vinegar and olive oil. If preferred, garnish with fresh basil and feta cheese. Warm or at room temperature, serve.

(If the quinoa and vegetables are pre-cooked, the prep time is 15 minutes.)

3. Wrapped Turkey or Tofurkey

Ingredients:
- lettuce leaves or whole-grain wrap
- Tofurkey (vegan option) or sliced turkey (non-vegan option).
- Avocado slices
- Tomato slices
- Greens, mixed
- Spreadable mustard or hummus

Instructions: Arrange the whole-grain wrap or lettuce leaves on a plate. Layer turkey or Tofurkey, avocado slices, tomatoes, and mixed greens on top. Spread mustard or hummus over top for extra flavor. Roll the wrap up and enjoy.

(Preparation time: 5 minutes)

4. Soup with lentils and vegetables

Ingredients:

- 1 cup lentils, cooked
- Vegetables (carrots, celery, onions, etc.)
- Broth of vegetables
- Fresh herbs (such as thyme and rosemary)
- Cooking with olive oil
- Season with salt and pepper to taste.

Instructions: Sauté mixed vegetables in olive oil in a saucepan until softened. Pour in the cooked lentils and vegetable broth. Season with salt, pepper, and fresh herbs. Simmer the vegetables until they are soft. Serve immediately.

(If the lentils are pre-cooked, the prep time is 20 minutes.)

5. Grilled Chicken or Tofu Salad with Greek Dressing

Ingredients:

- Tofu (for a vegan option) or grilled chicken breast
- Greens, mixed
- Cucumber slices, cherry tomatoes, and red onions
- The Kalamata olives
- Feta cheese or a dairy-free substitute
- Dressing: olive oil and balsamic vinegar
- Seasoning with oregano

Instructions: In a bowl, combine mixed greens, cucumbers, cherry tomatoes, red onions, and Kalamata olives. Serve with grilled chicken or tofu on top. Garnish with feta cheese (or a dairy-free substitute). Drizzle with olive oil, balsamic vinegar, and oregano to taste. Serve chilled.
(Preparation time: 15 minutes)

6. Bowl of Quinoa with Black Beans
Ingredients:
- 1 cup quinoa, cooked
- 1 pound black beans
- Red bell pepper, diced
- kernels of corn
- fresh cilantro, chopped

- Dressing: lime juice and olive oil
- Season with salt and pepper to taste.

Instructions: In a mixing bowl, combine cooked quinoa, black beans, red bell pepper, and corn kernels. Dress with lime juice and olive oil and toss with chopped cilantro. Season with salt and pepper to taste. At room temperature, serve.

(Preparation time: 10 minutes if the quinoa and beans are already cooked.)

7. Veggie and Hummus Wrap

Ingredients:
- lettuce leaves or whole-grain wrap
- Hummus (your favorite taste)
- Cucumbers, bell peppers, and carrots, sliced
- Greens, mixed
- Optional: sliced black olives

Instructions: Spread hummus generously on the whole-grain wrap or lettuce leaves. Sliced cucumbers, bell peppers, carrots, and mixed greens should be added. For added taste, sprinkle with sliced black olives. Roll the wrap up and enjoy.

(Preparation time: 5 minutes)

8. Salad with salmon or tempeh

Ingredients:

- Salmon, grilled or baked, or tempeh (for a vegan option).
- Greens, mixed
- Strawberries, sliced
- pecans or almonds, chopped
- **Dressing**: balsamic vinaigrette

Instructions: In a salad bowl, combine mixed greens, sliced strawberries, and chopped nuts. Serve with grilled or baked salmon or tempeh on top. Dress with the balsamic vinaigrette. Serve chilled.

(If the salmon or tempeh is already cooked, the prep time is 15 minutes.)

9. Stuffed Quinoa Bell Peppers

Ingredients:

- Cayenne peppers
- Quinoa simmered with vegetable broth
- Toasted tomatoes, diced
- spinach, finely chopped
- Crumbled feta cheese or a dairy-free substitute

- Basil leaves, fresh
- Drizzle with olive oil

Instructions: Preheat the oven to 375 degrees Fahrenheit (190 degrees Celsius). Remove the tops of the bell peppers and remove the seeds and membranes. Combine cooked quinoa, diced tomatoes, chopped spinach, and feta cheese (or dairy-free equivalent) in a mixing bowl. Stuff the quinoa mixture inside the bell peppers. Bake the filled peppers for 30-35 minutes in a baking dish drizzled with olive oil. Before serving, garnish with fresh basil leaves.

(Preparation time: 20 minutes if quinoa is already cooked)

10. Stir-Fry with Tofu and Vegetables
Ingredients:
- Cubed firm tofu
- Vegetables (broccoli, snap peas, bell peppers, etc.)
- Mushroom slices
- Green onions, sliced
- Soy sauce with low sodium or teriyaki sauce
- Stir-frying with olive oil

- Brown rice or quinoa, cooked

Instructions: In a wok or big skillet, heat the olive oil over medium-high heat. Stir in the cubed tofu until it turns golden. Set the tofu aside after removing it from the pan. Stir-fry the mixed vegetables and mushrooms in the same pan until tender. Return the tofu to the skillet and top with sliced green onions and low-sodium soy sauce or teriyaki sauce. Serve with brown rice or quinoa.

(Preparation time: 20 minutes)

Ten Dinner Options and How to Prepare Them

1. Lemon and Dill Baked Salmon

Ingredients:
- 2 fillets of salmon
- 1 sliced lemon
- Dill sprigs, fresh
- Extra virgin olive oil
- seasoned with salt & pepper

Instructions: Preheat the oven to 375 degrees Fahrenheit (190 degrees Celsius). Line a baking sheet with parchment paper

and place the salmon fillets on it. Season the salmon with salt and pepper and drizzle with olive oil. Garnish each fillet with lemon slices and dill sprigs. Bake the salmon for 15-20 minutes, or until it flakes easily with a fork. Serve immediately.
(Preparation time: 10 minutes)

2. Stir-Fry of Quinoa and Vegetables
Ingredients:
- 1 cup quinoa, cooked
- Vegetables (such as bell peppers, broccoli, and carrots)
- Mushroom slices
- Snap peas or snow peas?
- Green onions, sliced
- Soy sauce with low sodium or teriyaki sauce
- Stir-frying with olive oil

Instructions: In a wok or big skillet, heat the olive oil over medium-high heat. Mix in the veggies, mushrooms, snow peas, and green onions, if using. Stir-fry the vegetables until they are soft. Drizzle with low-sodium soy sauce or teriyaki sauce and top with cooked quinoa. Cook for a further 2-3 minutes after tossing everything together. Serve immediately.

(Preparation time: 20 minutes if quinoa is already cooked)

3. Kebabs with chicken or tofu and vegetables

Ingredients:

- Cubes of chicken breast or tofu
- Red onions, bell peppers, and zucchini (cut into bits)
- Extra virgin olive oil
- Juice of lemon
- Garlic, Oregano, and Thyme
- Water-soaked wooden skewers

Instructions: Combine the olive oil, lemon juice, minced garlic, oregano, and thyme in a mixing bowl. Thread the moistened wooden skewers with the chicken or tofu and vegetables. Brush the chicken with the olive oil mixture. Grill or bake the kebabs until thoroughly done. Serve immediately.

(Time to prepare: 20 minutes, plus grilling or baking time)

4. Pesto Spaghetti Squash

Ingredients:

- 1 spaghetti squash Pesto sauce (homemade or store-bought) (check ingredients for A+ compatibility)
- Basil leaves, fresh
- Optional: grated Parmesan cheese or dairy-free substitute

Instructions: Preheat the oven to 375 degrees Fahrenheit (190 degrees Celsius). Remove the seeds from the spaghetti squash and cut it in half lengthwise. Place the squash halves on a baking sheet, cut side down, and bake for 30-40 minutes, or until soft. Scrape the flesh into "spaghetti" strands with a fork. Toss with pesto sauce and serve with fresh basil on top. If preferred, top with grated Parmesan cheese or a dairy-free substitute. Serve hot.

(Time to prepare: 10 minutes, plus baking time)

5. Curry with lentils and vegetables

Ingredients:

- 1 cup lentils, cooked
- Vegetables (such as bell peppers, carrots, and zucchini)

- Coconut cream
- Curry paste (confirm A+ compatibility with the ingredients)
- Extra virgin olive oil
- cilantro leaves, fresh
- seasoned with salt & pepper

Instructions: Warm the olive oil in a large saucepan over medium heat. Sauté the mixed vegetables until they are slightly soft. Incorporate the cooked lentils and curry paste. Pour in the coconut milk and heat until the vegetables are tender. Season with salt and pepper to taste. Garnish with fresh cilantro leaves if desired. Serve alongside rice or quinoa.

(If the lentils are pre-cooked, the prep time is 20 minutes.)

6. Tofu Stir-Fried with Broccoli and Cashews

Ingredients:
- Tofu (cubed)
- Florets of broccoli
- Cashews
- Garlic, minced Ginger, olive oil, soy sauce or tamari

Instructions: In a wok or big skillet, heat the olive oil over medium-high heat. Stir in the cubed tofu until it turns golden. Set the tofu aside after removing it from the pan. Stir-fry broccoli florets, minced garlic, and minced ginger in the same pan until soft. Return the tofu to the pan and stir in the cashews. Drizzle with soy sauce or tamari to taste. Over brown rice or quinoa, serve. **(Preparation time: 20 minutes)**

7. Pesto Zucchini Noodles with Cherry Tomatoes

Ingredients:

- Spiralized zucchini noodles
- Pesto sauce, homemade or purchased (check components for A+ compatibility)
- halved cherry tomatoes, roasted pine nuts (optional)

Instructions: Sauté zucchini noodles in a large skillet until just tender. Toss with pesto sauce and half cherry tomatoes. If preferred, top with toasted pine nuts. Serve hot. **(Preparation time: 10 minutes)**

8. Portobello Mushrooms with Quinoa Grilled

Ingredients:

- Portobello mushrooms, washed and de-stemmed
- Extra virgin olive oil
- Vinegar of Modena
- Quinoa has been cooked.
- fresh parsley, chopped
- seasoned with salt & pepper

Instructions: Preheat the grill to medium-high temperature. Combine the olive oil and balsamic vinegar in a mixing basin. Brush the oil and vinegar mixture over the mushroom tops. Grill the mushrooms for 4-5 minutes per side, or until they are soft. Garnish with chopped fresh parsley and serve over cooked quinoa. Season with salt and pepper to taste. Serve immediately.

(Preparation time: 15 minutes)

9. Chicken or Tempeh Stir-Fry with Asparagus and Snap Peas

Ingredients:

- Asparagus, chopped into bits, sliced chicken breast or tempeh

- Peas, snap
- Garlic, minced Ginger, olive oil, low-sodium soy sauce or tamari

Instructions: In a wok or big skillet, heat the olive oil over medium-high heat. Cook until the chicken or tempeh is done. Set aside after removing from the pan. Stir-fry the asparagus and snap peas in the same pan until tender-crisp. Put the chicken or tempeh back in the pan. Drizzle with tamari or low-sodium soy sauce. Over brown rice or quinoa, serve.

(Preparation time: 20 minutes)

10. Lasagna with Eggplant & Zucchini (Vegan)

Ingredients:

- Thinly sliced lengthwise eggplant and zucchini
- Tomato sauce (confirm that the ingredients are A+ compatible)
- Ricotta cheese (vegan or dairy-based if desired)
- Basil leaves, fresh
- Extra virgin olive oil
- seasoned with salt & pepper

Instructions: Preheat the oven to 375 degrees Fahrenheit (190 degrees Celsius). Layer eggplant and zucchini slices, tomato sauce, and vegan ricotta cheese (or dairy-based) in a baking dish. Drizzle with olive oil and top with fresh basil leaves. Season with salt and pepper to taste. Layers should be repeated. Bake the vegetables for 30-40 minutes, or until tender. Serve immediately.

(Preparation time: 20 minutes)

Ten Snacks And Appetizers and How to Prepare Them

1. Bites of cucumber and hummus
Ingredients:
- Slices of cucumber
- Check the ingredients for A+ compatibility before making hummus.
- Tomatoes in the shape of cherries
- Basil leaves, fresh
- Drizzle with olive oil and balsamic vinegar
- seasoned with salt & pepper

Instructions: Dollop hummus on top of each cucumber slice. On top, place a half cherry tomato. Serve with a fresh basil leaf as a garnish. Drizzle with balsamic vinegar and olive oil. Season with salt and pepper to taste. Serve chilled.
(Preparation time: 10 minutes)

2. Guacamole with Carrot Sticks
Ingredients:
- Avocados that have matured
- Juice of lime
- finely sliced red onion
- chopped fresh cilantro
- Toasted tomatoes, diced
- Jalapeo pepper (optional, for extra heat)
- Veggie sticks (carrots, bell peppers, celery, etc.)

Instructions: Mash the ripe avocados with the lime juice. Stir in the chopped red onion, fresh cilantro, diced tomatoes, and finely chopped jalapeo pepper, if using. Serve with a variety of vegetable sticks. Serve chilled.
(Preparation time: 15 minutes)

3. Skewers of Greek Salad

Ingredients:
- Tomatoes in the shape of cherries
- Cucumber slices
- The Kalamata olives
- Feta cheese or a dairy-free substitute (confirm A+ compatibility with the ingredients)
- Basil leaves, fresh
- Drizzle with olive oil and balsamic vinegar
- seasoned with salt & pepper

Instructions: Thread skewers with cherry tomatoes, cucumber slices, Kalamata olives, and cubes of feta cheese or a dairy-free substitute. Garnish with fresh basil leaves if desired. Drizzle with balsamic vinegar and olive oil. Season with salt and pepper to taste. Serve chilled.

(Preparation time: 15 minutes)

4. Banana Slices and Almond Butter

Ingredients:
- Bananas, cut into slices
- The almond butter
- Optional chopped almonds

- Optional cinnamon

Instructions: On each banana slice, spread a tiny amount of almond butter. If preferred, top with sliced almonds and a pinch of cinnamon. Serve right away.

(Preparation time: 5 minutes)

5. Avocado and tomato rice cakes
Ingredients:
- Rice cakes (confirm that the components are A+ compatible)
- Avocados that have matured
- Tomato slices
- Drizzle with olive oil and balsamic vinegar
- seasoned with salt & pepper

Instructions: Each rice cake should be topped with mashed ripe avocado and sliced tomatoes. Drizzle with balsamic vinegar and olive oil. Season with salt and pepper to taste. Serve right away.

(Preparation time: 10 minutes)

6. Hummus with Roasted Red Peppers
Ingredients:

- Roasted red peppers, canned or jarred (check ingredients for A+ compatibility)
- Chickpeas
- Juice of lemon
- Garlic, Tahini, minced (check ingredients for A+ compatibility)
- Extra virgin olive oil
- Optional paprika and cayenne pepper
- For dipping, use veggie sticks, pita chips, or rice cakes.

Instructions: Combine roasted red peppers, chickpeas, lemon juice, minced garlic, tahini, and olive oil in a food processor. If desired, season with paprika and cayenne pepper. Blend until completely smooth. Dip with vegetable sticks, pita chips, or rice cakes. Serve chilled.

(Preparation time: 15 minutes)

7. Salad with Fresh Fruits

Ingredients:
- A variety of A+ fruit (for example, blueberries, strawberries, kiwi, and apples)
- Mint leaves, fresh

- Juice of lemon
- **Optional:** honey or maple syrup

Instructions: Wash the fruits, peel them, and cut them into bite-sized pieces. In a mixing bowl, combine the fruits. To keep the fruit fresh, sprinkle it with lemon juice. If you want to add more sweetness, drizzle with honey or maple syrup. Garnish with fresh mint leaves if desired. Serve chilled.
(Preparation time: 10 minutes)

8. Sweet Potato Fries Baked
Ingredients:
- Cut sweet potatoes into fry
- Optional: olive oil, paprika, and rosemary
- seasoned with salt & pepper

Instructions: Preheat the oven to 425 degrees Fahrenheit (220 degrees Celsius). Season the sweet potato fries with paprika, rosemary, salt, and pepper after tossing them in olive oil. Place them in a single layer on a baking pan. Bake for 20 to 25 minutes, or until crispy and golden. Serve immediately.
(Preparation time: 15 minutes)

9. Apples sliced with almond butter and cinnamon

Ingredients:

- Apple slices
- The almond butter
- a dash of cinnamon

Instructions: On each apple slice, spread almond butter. Garnish with a pinch of cinnamon. Serve right away.

(Preparation time: 5 minutes)

10. Caprese Skewers

Ingredients:

- Tomatoes in the shape of cherries
- Fresh mozzarella or a dairy-free substitute (for A+ compatibility, check the ingredients)
- Basil leaves, fresh
- Drizzle with olive oil and balsamic vinegar
- seasoned with salt & pepper

Instructions: Thread skewers with cherry tomatoes, mozzarella (or a dairy-free substitute), and fresh basil leaves. Drizzle with balsamic vinegar and olive oil. Season with salt and pepper to taste. Serve chilled.

(Preparation time: 10 minutes)

Ten Desserts and Ho to Prepare Them

1. Berries and Chia Seed Pudding

Ingredients:

- 2 tbsp of chia seeds
- 1 cup almond milk (or a dairy-free substitute)
- a half teaspoon of vanilla extract
- Optional: 1 tablespoon honey or maple syrup
- Topping: mixed berries

Instructions: Combine the chia seeds, almond milk, and vanilla essence in a mixing dish. If desired, sweeten with honey or maple syrup. Stir thoroughly and place in the refrigerator for several hours or overnight to thicken. Garnish with mixed berries. Serve chilled.

(Preparation time: 5 minutes plus rest time)

2. Almond and Berry Pudding

Ingredients:

- Almond yogurt (for A+ compatibility, verify the ingredients)
- Berries in a variety of colors
- Almonds, optionally chopped honey or maple syrup

Instructions: Layer almond yogurt, mixed berries, and sliced almonds in a glass or bowl. If desired, drizzle with honey or maple syrup. Repeat for a second layer. With a spoon, serve.

(Preparation time: 5 minutes)

3. Cinnamon-Baked Apples

Ingredients:
- halved and cored apples
- Cinnamon
- Optional chopped walnuts or pecans
- **Optional:** honey or maple syrup

Instructions: Preheat the oven to 375 degrees Fahrenheit (190 degrees Celsius). Place apple halves cut side up in a baking dish. If desired, top with cinnamon and chopped nuts. If you like more sweetness, drizzle with honey or maple syrup. Bake the apples for 30-40 minutes, or until soft. Serve hot.

(Time to prepare: 10 minutes, plus baking time)

4. Bites with banana and almond butter
Ingredients:
- Bananas cut into rounds
- The almond butter
- Optional unsweetened shredded coconut
- Chips in dark chocolate (Confirm that the ingredients are A+ compatible.)

Instructions: On each banana slice, spread a tiny amount of almond butter. Finish with shredded coconut and a dark chocolate chip. Serve right away.

(Preparation time: 5 minutes)

5. Salad with Berries and Nuts
Ingredients:
- Berries (strawberries, blueberries, raspberries, etc.)
- Chopped mixed nuts (almonds, walnuts, pecans, etc.)
- Mint leaves, fresh
- **Optional:** honey or maple syrup

Instructions: In a mixing bowl, combine mixed berries and chopped mixed nuts. Garnish with fresh mint leaves if desired. If desired, drizzle with honey or maple syrup. Serve chilled.

(Preparation time: 10 minutes)

6. Mousse de Chocolate et Avocado
Ingredients:
- Avocados that have matured
- Cocoa (unsweetened) powder
- Maple or honey syrup
- Vanilla flavoring
- a grain of salt

Instructions: Combine ripe avocados, cocoa powder, honey or maple syrup, vanilla essence, and a bit of salt in a blender or food processor. Blend until the mixture is smooth and creamy. Refrigerate for at least 30 minutes prior to serving. Serve chilled.

(Preparation time: 10 minutes)

7. Banana Popsicle
Ingredients:
- Half-cut bananas in Greek yogurt (or dairy-free substitute)

- Chopped nuts (almonds, pecans, etc.)
- Check the components for A+ compatibility before using dark chocolate chips.
- Popsicle sticks made of wood

Instructions: Insert a wooden popsicle stick into either half of a banana. Dip each banana in Greek yogurt, allowing excess to drip off. Chopped nuts and dark chocolate chips are optional. Place on a baking sheet and place in the freezer until solid. Serve cold.

(Time to prepare: 15 minutes, including freezing time)

8. Baked Spiced Pears
Ingredients:
- halved and cored pears
- Nutmeg and cinnamon
- Almonds or walnuts, chopped
- Optional: honey or maple syrup

Instructions: Preheat the oven to 375 degrees Fahrenheit (190 degrees Celsius). Place pear halves cut side up in a baking dish. Season with cinnamon, nutmeg, and chopped nuts to taste. If you like more sweetness, drizzle with honey or maple syrup. Bake the pears for 30-40 minutes, or until they are soft. Serve hot.

(*Time to prepare*: **10 minutes, plus baking time**)

9. Roll-Ups with Fruit and Nut Butter

Ingredients:
- Tortillas made from whole grains (A+ option)
- Cashew or almond butter
- Bananas or strawberries, sliced
- Chopped nuts (almonds, walnuts, etc.)
- *Optional*: honey or maple syrup

Instructions: In a dry skillet, warm the whole-grain tortilla gently. Spread the tortilla with almond or cashew butter. Arrange sliced bananas or strawberries on a platter and top with chopped almonds. If desired, drizzle with honey or maple syrup. Roll it up and eat it.

(*Preparation time: 5 minutes*)

10. Sorbet with fresh mint and lemon

Ingredients:
- Mint leaves, fresh
- Juice of lemon

- Maple or honey syrup

Instructions: Blend together fresh mint leaves, lemon juice, honey or maple syrup, and water in a blender. Blend until everything is well incorporated. Fill an ice cream maker halfway with the ingredients and churn until it achieves a sorbet-like consistency. Alternatively, spoon the mixture into a shallow dish and freeze until hard, stirring every 30 minutes. Serve chilled.

(Time to prepare: 15 minutes, including freezing time)

Ten Smoothies and How to Prepare Them

1. Smoothie with Berries
Ingredients:
- 1 cup berries (strawberries, blueberries, raspberries, etc.)
- a half banana
- 1 cup almond milk (or dairy-free substitute)
- 1 teaspoon chia seeds

- Optional: honey or maple syrup for sweetness

Instructions: Blend till smooth the mixed berries, banana, almond milk, and chia seeds. If desired, sweeten with honey or maple syrup. Serve chilled.

(Preparation time: 5 minutes)

2. Smoothie with Green Goodness

Ingredients:

- 1 pound spinach
- a half avocado
- a half banana
- 1 cup almond milk (or dairy-free substitute)
- 1 tablespoon flaxseed meal
- **Optional:** honey or maple syrup for sweetness

Instructions: Smoothly combine spinach, avocado, banana, almond milk, and ground flaxseed. If desired, sweeten with honey or maple syrup. Serve chilled.

(Preparation time: 5 minutes)

3. Smoothie with Pineapple Paradise

Ingredients:

- 1 cup pineapple chunks, fresh or frozen
- a half banana
- 1/2 cup coconut milk (or a dairy-free substitute)
- 1 tbsp. shredded coconut
- Optional: honey or maple syrup for sweetness

Instructions: Smoothly combine pineapple pieces, banana, coconut milk, and shredded coconut. If desired, sweeten with honey or maple syrup. Serve chilled.

(Preparation time: 5 minutes)

4. Smoothie with Tropical Turmeric
Ingredients:
- 1 cup fresh or frozen mango chunks
- a half banana
- 1 cup of coconut water
- 1 tablespoon turmeric powder
- a pinch of black pepper (to aid in the absorption of turmeric)
- **Optional:** honey or maple syrup for sweetness

Instructions: Smoothly combine mango pieces, banana, coconut water, turmeric powder, and black pepper. If desired, sweeten with honey or maple syrup. Serve chilled.

(Preparation time: 5 minutes)

5. Smoothie with Blueberries and Almonds

Ingredients:
- 1 cup fresh or frozen blueberries
- a half banana
- 1 cup almond milk (or dairy-free substitute)
- 1 tbsp. almond butter
- Optional: honey or maple syrup for sweetness

Instructions: Blueberries, banana, almond milk, and almond butter should be blended till smooth. If desired, sweeten with honey or maple syrup. Serve chilled.

(Preparation time: 5 minutes)

6. Smoothie with beets and berries

Ingredients:
- 1 small peeled and chopped cooked beet
- 1/2 cup mixed berries (strawberries, blueberries, etc.)

- a half banana
- 1 cup almond milk (or dairy-free substitute)
- Optional: honey or maple syrup for sweetness

Instructions: Blend until smooth cooked beet, mixed berries, banana, and almond milk. If desired, sweeten with honey or maple syrup. Serve chilled.

(Preparation time: 5 minutes)

7. Smoothie with Carrot Cake

Ingredients:
- 1 peeled and sliced carrot
- a half banana
- 1 cup almond milk (or dairy-free substitute)
- 1/4 teaspoon cinnamon powder
- a dash of nutmeg
- Optional: honey or maple syrup for sweetness

Instructions: Blend carrot, banana, almond milk, cinnamon, and nutmeg together until creamy. If desired, sweeten with honey or maple syrup. Serve chilled.

(Preparation time: 5 minutes)

8. Smoothie with Kiwi and Spinach

Ingredients:

- 2 peeled and sliced kiwis
- 1 pound spinach
- a half banana
- 1 cup almond milk (or dairy-free substitute)
- Optional: honey or maple syrup for sweetness

Instructions: Blend together the kiwis, spinach, banana, and almond milk until smooth. If desired, sweeten with honey or maple syrup. Serve chilled.

(Preparation time: 5 minutes)

9. Smoothie with pears and ginger

Ingredients:

- 1 peeled and diced ripe pear
- a half banana
- 1 cup almond milk (or dairy-free substitute)
- 1/2 inch fresh ginger, peeled and chopped
- Optional: honey or maple syrup for sweetness

Instructions: Blend till smooth the ripe pear, banana, almond milk, and fresh ginger. If desired, sweeten with honey or maple syrup. Serve chilled.

(Preparation time: 5 minutes)

10. Smoothie with Chocolate and Almonds
Ingredients:
- 1 tbsp. unsweetened cocoa powder
- a half banana
- 1 cup almond milk (or a dairy-free substitute)
- 1 tbsp. almond butter
- Optional: honey or maple syrup for sweetness

Instructions: Smoothly combine cocoa powder, banana, almond milk, and almond butter. If desired, sweeten with honey or maple syrup. Serve chilled.

(Preparation time: 5 minutes)

Note: Depending on your nutritional needs and tastes, modify the ingredients and portion quantities as necessary. Enjoy your nutritious and delicious meals all week long!

Enjoy!

CONCLUSIONS

As you finish the A+ Blood Type Diet book, I want to underline that you have power over your health and well-being. Your understanding of how your blood type affects your dietary choices is a great weapon. You may take ownership of your health and experience the transformative impacts of eating in harmony with your body's demands by accepting this concept and applying the methods provided in this book.

The A+ Blood Type Diet is a way of life that promotes vitality, wellbeing, and longevity. Remember that even little modifications in your everyday food choices can lead to substantial gains in your health. You nourish your body in the most tailored and effective way possible by eating foods that match your blood type.

I encourage you to keep researching, experimenting, and enjoying the tasty and healthful dishes in this book. Allow this knowledge to enable you to make informed decisions, laying the groundwork for a healthier and more vibrant future. Accept the A+ Blood Type Diet and live a life of better health, more energy, and long-term well-being. Your journey to a healthy you begins here.

My Little Request

Dear valued customer, if you've enjoyed my **Blood Type A+ Diet book**, *I kindly request you to please take a moment to rate it with five stars (★★★★★) on Amazon and share a positive review. Your feedback is greatly appreciated as it motivates me to write more quality books.*

Thanks!

Journals to Plan Your Diet

A+ FOODS PLANNER

			GROCERY LIST
MONDAY	BREAKFAST		
	LUNCH		
	DINNER		
TUESDAY	BREAKFAST		
	LUNCH		
	DINNER		
WEDNESDAY	BREAKFAST		
	LUNCH		
	DINNER		
THURSDAY	BREAKFAST		
	LUNCH		
	DINNER		
FRIDAY	BREAKFAST		
	LUNCH		SNACKS
	DINNER		
SATURDAY	BREAKFAST		
	LUNCH		
	DINNER		
SUNDAY	BREAKFAST		
	LUNCH		
	DINNER		

A+ FOODS PLANNER

MONDAY	BREAKFAST	
	LUNCH	
	DINNER	
TUESDAY	BREAKFAST	
	LUNCH	
	DINNER	
WEDNESDAY	BREAKFAST	
	LUNCH	
	DINNER	
THURSDAY	BREAKFAST	
	LUNCH	
	DINNER	
FRIDAY	BREAKFAST	
	LUNCH	
	DINNER	
SATURDAY	BREAKFAST	
	LUNCH	
	DINNER	
SUNDAY	BREAKFAST	
	LUNCH	
	DINNER	

GROCERY LIST

_____
_____
_____
_____
_____
_____
_____
_____
_____

SNACKS

_____
_____
_____
_____

A+ FOODS PLANNER

			GROCERY LIST
MONDAY	BREAKFAST		
	LUNCH		
	DINNER		
TUESDAY	BREAKFAST		
	LUNCH		
	DINNER		
WEDNESDAY	BREAKFAST		
	LUNCH		
	DINNER		
THURSDAY	BREAKFAST		
	LUNCH		
	DINNER		
FRIDAY	BREAKFAST		
	LUNCH		SNACKS
	DINNER		
SATURDAY	BREAKFAST		
	LUNCH		
	DINNER		
SUNDAY	BREAKFAST		
	LUNCH		
	DINNER		

A+ FOODS PLANNER

			GROCERY LIST
MONDAY	BREAKFAST		
	LUNCH		
	DINNER		
TUESDAY	BREAKFAST		
	LUNCH		
	DINNER		
WEDNESDAY	BREAKFAST		
	LUNCH		
	DINNER		
THURSDAY	BREAKFAST		
	LUNCH		
	DINNER		
FRIDAY	BREAKFAST		
	LUNCH		SNACKS
	DINNER		
SATURDAY	BREAKFAST		
	LUNCH		
	DINNER		
SUNDAY	BREAKFAST		
	LUNCH		
	DINNER		

A+ FOODS PLANNER

			GROCERY LIST
MONDAY	BREAKFAST		
	LUNCH		
	DINNER		
TUESDAY	BREAKFAST		
	LUNCH		
	DINNER		
WEDNESDAY	BREAKFAST		
	LUNCH		
	DINNER		
THURSDAY	BREAKFAST		
	LUNCH		
	DINNER		
FRIDAY	BREAKFAST		SNACKS
	LUNCH		
	DINNER		
SATURDAY	BREAKFAST		
	LUNCH		
	DINNER		
SUNDAY	BREAKFAST		
	LUNCH		
	DINNER		

A+ FOODS PLANNER

			GROCERY LIST
MONDAY	BREAKFAST		
	LUNCH		_____
	DINNER		_____
TUESDAY	BREAKFAST		_____
	LUNCH		_____
	DINNER		_____
WEDNESDAY	BREAKFAST		_____
	LUNCH		_____
	DINNER		_____
THURSDAY	BREAKFAST		_____
	LUNCH		_____
	DINNER		_____
FRIDAY	BREAKFAST		
	LUNCH		SNACKS
	DINNER		
SATURDAY	BREAKFAST		_____
	LUNCH		_____
	DINNER		_____
SUNDAY	BREAKFAST		_____
	LUNCH		_____
	DINNER		_____

A+ FOODS PLANNER

			GROCERY LIST
MONDAY	BREAKFAST		
	LUNCH		
	DINNER		
TUESDAY	BREAKFAST		
	LUNCH		
	DINNER		
WEDNESDAY	BREAKFAST		
	LUNCH		
	DINNER		
THURSDAY	BREAKFAST		
	LUNCH		
	DINNER		
FRIDAY	BREAKFAST		SNACKS
	LUNCH		
	DINNER		
SATURDAY	BREAKFAST		
	LUNCH		
	DINNER		
SUNDAY	BREAKFAST		
	LUNCH		
	DINNER		

A+ FOODS PLANNER

			GROCERY LIST
MONDAY	BREAKFAST		
	LUNCH		
	DINNER		
TUESDAY	BREAKFAST		
	LUNCH		
	DINNER		
WEDNESDAY	BREAKFAST		
	LUNCH		
	DINNER		
THURSDAY	BREAKFAST		
	LUNCH		
	DINNER		
FRIDAY	BREAKFAST		SNACKS
	LUNCH		
	DINNER		
SATURDAY	BREAKFAST		
	LUNCH		
	DINNER		
SUNDAY	BREAKFAST		
	LUNCH		
	DINNER		

A+ FOODS PLANNER

MONDAY	BREAKFAST		**GROCERY LIST**
	LUNCH		
	DINNER		
TUESDAY	BREAKFAST		
	LUNCH		
	DINNER		
WEDNESDAY	BREAKFAST		
	LUNCH		
	DINNER		
THURSDAY	BREAKFAST		
	LUNCH		
	DINNER		
FRIDAY	BREAKFAST		
	LUNCH		**SNACKS**
	DINNER		
SATURDAY	BREAKFAST		
	LUNCH		
	DINNER		
SUNDAY	BREAKFAST		
	LUNCH		
	DINNER		

A+ FOODS PLANNER

			GROCERY LIST
MONDAY	BREAKFAST		
	LUNCH		
	DINNER		
TUESDAY	BREAKFAST		
	LUNCH		
	DINNER		
WEDNESDAY	BREAKFAST		
	LUNCH		
	DINNER		
THURSDAY	BREAKFAST		
	LUNCH		
	DINNER		
FRIDAY	BREAKFAST		
	LUNCH		SNACKS
	DINNER		
SATURDAY	BREAKFAST		
	LUNCH		
	DINNER		
SUNDAY	BREAKFAST		
	LUNCH		
	DINNER		

A+ FOODS PLANNER

			GROCERY LIST
MONDAY	BREAKFAST		
	LUNCH		
	DINNER		
TUESDAY	BREAKFAST		
	LUNCH		
	DINNER		
WEDNESDAY	BREAKFAST		
	LUNCH		
	DINNER		
THURSDAY	BREAKFAST		
	LUNCH		
	DINNER		
FRIDAY	BREAKFAST		SNACKS
	LUNCH		
	DINNER		
SATURDAY	BREAKFAST		
	LUNCH		
	DINNER		
SUNDAY	BREAKFAST		
	LUNCH		
	DINNER		

A+ FOODS PLANNER

				GROCERY LIST
MONDAY	BREAKFAST			_____
	LUNCH			_____
	DINNER			_____
TUESDAY	BREAKFAST			_____
	LUNCH			_____
	DINNER			_____
WEDNESDAY	BREAKFAST			_____
	LUNCH			_____
	DINNER			_____
THURSDAY	BREAKFAST			_____
	LUNCH			_____
	DINNER			
FRIDAY	BREAKFAST			SNACKS
	LUNCH			_____
	DINNER			_____
SATURDAY	BREAKFAST			_____
	LUNCH			_____
	DINNER			_____
SUNDAY	BREAKFAST			_____
	LUNCH			_____
	DINNER			

A+ FOODS PLANNER

			GROCERY LIST
MONDAY	BREAKFAST		
	LUNCH		_____
	DINNER		_____
TUESDAY	BREAKFAST		_____
	LUNCH		_____
	DINNER		_____
WEDNESDAY	BREAKFAST		_____
	LUNCH		_____
	DINNER		_____
THURSDAY	BREAKFAST		_____
	LUNCH		_____
	DINNER		_____
FRIDAY	BREAKFAST		SNACKS
	LUNCH		
	DINNER		_____
SATURDAY	BREAKFAST		_____
	LUNCH		_____
	DINNER		_____
SUNDAY	BREAKFAST		_____
	LUNCH		_____
	DINNER		_____

A+ FOODS PLANNER

			GROCERY LIST
MONDAY	BREAKFAST		
	LUNCH		————
	DINNER		————
TUESDAY	BREAKFAST		————
	LUNCH		————
	DINNER		————
WEDNESDAY	BREAKFAST		————
	LUNCH		————
	DINNER		————
THURSDAY	BREAKFAST		————
	LUNCH		————
	DINNER		————
FRIDAY	BREAKFAST		
	LUNCH		**SNACKS**
	DINNER		
SATURDAY	BREAKFAST		————
	LUNCH		————
	DINNER		————
SUNDAY	BREAKFAST		————
	LUNCH		————
	DINNER		

A+ FOODS PLANNER

			GROCERY LIST
MONDAY	BREAKFAST		
	LUNCH		_____
	DINNER		_____
TUESDAY	BREAKFAST		_____
	LUNCH		_____
	DINNER		_____
WEDNESDAY	BREAKFAST		_____
	LUNCH		_____
	DINNER		_____
THURSDAY	BREAKFAST		_____
	LUNCH		_____
	DINNER		_____

			SNACKS
FRIDAY	BREAKFAST		
	LUNCH		_____
	DINNER		_____
SATURDAY	BREAKFAST		_____
	LUNCH		_____
	DINNER		_____
SUNDAY	BREAKFAST		_____
	LUNCH		_____
	DINNER		

A+ FOODS PLANNER

			GROCERY LIST
MONDAY	BREAKFAST		
	LUNCH		
	DINNER		
TUESDAY	BREAKFAST		
	LUNCH		
	DINNER		
WEDNESDAY	BREAKFAST		
	LUNCH		
	DINNER		
THURSDAY	BREAKFAST		
	LUNCH		
	DINNER		
FRIDAY	BREAKFAST		SNACKS
	LUNCH		
	DINNER		
SATURDAY	BREAKFAST		
	LUNCH		
	DINNER		
SUNDAY	BREAKFAST		
	LUNCH		
	DINNER		

A+ FOODS PLANNER

			GROCERY LIST
MONDAY	BREAKFAST		
	LUNCH		
	DINNER		
TUESDAY	BREAKFAST		
	LUNCH		
	DINNER		
WEDNESDAY	BREAKFAST		
	LUNCH		
	DINNER		
THURSDAY	BREAKFAST		
	LUNCH		
	DINNER		
FRIDAY	BREAKFAST		SNACKS
	LUNCH		
	DINNER		
SATURDAY	BREAKFAST		
	LUNCH		
	DINNER		
SUNDAY	BREAKFAST		
	LUNCH		
	DINNER		

A+ FOODS PLANNER

			GROCERY LIST
MONDAY	BREAKFAST		
	LUNCH		
	DINNER		
TUESDAY	BREAKFAST		
	LUNCH		
	DINNER		
WEDNESDAY	BREAKFAST		
	LUNCH		
	DINNER		
THURSDAY	BREAKFAST		
	LUNCH		
	DINNER		
FRIDAY	BREAKFAST		
	LUNCH		SNACKS
	DINNER		
SATURDAY	BREAKFAST		
	LUNCH		
	DINNER		
SUNDAY	BREAKFAST		
	LUNCH		
	DINNER		

A+ FOODS PLANNER

			GROCERY LIST
MONDAY	BREAKFAST		
	LUNCH		
	DINNER		
TUESDAY	BREAKFAST		
	LUNCH		
	DINNER		
WEDNESDAY	BREAKFAST		
	LUNCH		
	DINNER		
THURSDAY	BREAKFAST		
	LUNCH		
	DINNER		
FRIDAY	BREAKFAST		SNACKS
	LUNCH		
	DINNER		
SATURDAY	BREAKFAST		
	LUNCH		
	DINNER		
SUNDAY	BREAKFAST		
	LUNCH		
	DINNER		

A+ FOODS PLANNER

				GROCERY LIST
MONDAY	BREAKFAST			
	LUNCH			_____
	DINNER			_____
TUESDAY	BREAKFAST			_____
	LUNCH			_____
	DINNER			_____
WEDNESDAY	BREAKFAST			_____
	LUNCH			_____
	DINNER			_____
THURSDAY	BREAKFAST			_____
	LUNCH			_____
	DINNER			_____
FRIDAY	BREAKFAST			SNACKS
	LUNCH			_____
	DINNER			_____
SATURDAY	BREAKFAST			_____
	LUNCH			_____
	DINNER			_____
SUNDAY	BREAKFAST			_____
	LUNCH			
	DINNER			

Printed in Dunstable, United Kingdom